BHAKTI YOGA

BHAKTI YOGA

SWAMI VIVEKANANDA

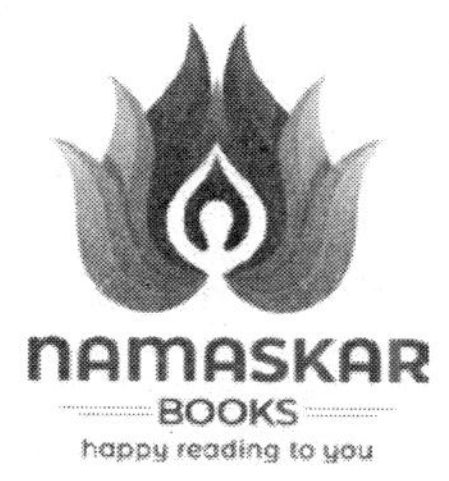

Published by
NAMASKAR BOOKS
Building No. 2/42 (Second Floor)
Ansari Road, Daryaganj
New Delhi-110002
e-mail: namaskarbooks@gmail.com
Website: www.namaskarbooks.com

ISBN: 978-93-5571-582-1

Bhakti Yoga
By Swami Vivekanand

Edition 2026

Price
₹ 150.00 (Rupees One Hundred Fifty only)

Printed at R-Tech Offset Printers, Delhi

Contents

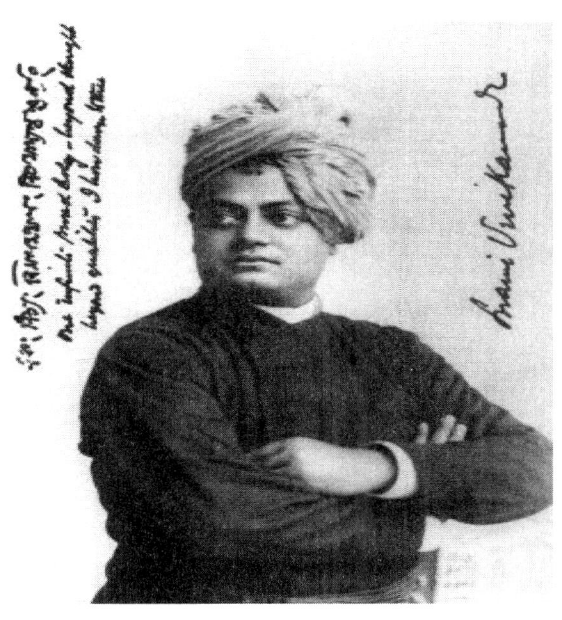

Based on lectures the Swami delivered in his rented rooms at 228 W 39th Street in December, 1895 and January, 1896. The classes were free of charge. Generally the Swami held two classes daily- morning and evening.

Although the Swami delivered many lectures and held numerous classes in the two years and five months he had been in America, these lectures constituted a departure in the way they were recorded. Just prior to the commencement of his Winter -95-96 season in NYC, his friends and supporters aided him by advertising for and ultimately hiring a professional stenographer: The man selected, Joseph Josiah Goodwin, later became a disciple of the Swami and followed him to England and India.

Four Paths of Yoga

(Written by the Swami during his first visit to America in answer to questions put by a Western disciple.)

Our main problem is to be free. It is evident then that until we realise ourselves as the Absolute, we cannot attain to deliverance. Yet there are various ways of attaining to this realisation. These methods have the generic name of Yoga (to join, to join ourselves to our reality). These Yogas, though divided into various groups, can principally be classed into four; and as each is only a method leading indirectly to the realisation of the Absolute, they are suited to different temperaments. Now it must be remembered that it is not that the assumed man becomes the real man or Absolute. There is no becoming with the Absolute. It is ever free, ever perfect; but the ignorance that has covered Its nature for a time is to be removed. Therefore the whole scope of all systems of Yoga (and each religion represents one) is to clear up this ignorance and allow the Âtman to restore its own nature. The chief helps in this liberation are Abhyâsa and Vairâgya.

Vairagya is non-attachment to life, because it is the will to enjoy that brings all this bondage in its train; and Abhyasa is constant practice of any one of the Yogas.

Karma Yoga. Karma Yoga is purifying the mind by means of work. Now if any work is done, good or bad, it must produce as a result a good or bad effect; no power can stay it, once the cause is present. Therefore good action producing good Karma, and bad action, bad Karma, the soul will go on in eternal bondage without ever hoping for deliverance. Now Karma belongs only to the body or the mind, never to the Atman (Self); only it can cast a veil before the Atman. The veil cast by bad Karma is ignorance. Good Karma has the power to strengthen the moral powers. And thus it creates non-attachment; it destroys the tendency towards bad Karma and thereby purifies the mind. But if the work is done with the intention of enjoyment, it then produces only that very enjoyment and does not purify the mind or Chitta. Therefore all work should be done without any desire to enjoy the fruits thereof. All fear and all desire to enjoy here or hereafter must be banished for ever by the Karma-Yogi. Moreover, this Karma without desire of return will destroy the selfishness, which is the root of all bondage. The watchword of the Karma-Yogi is "not I, but Thou", and no amount of self-sacrifice is too much for him. But he does this without any desire to go to heaven, or gain name or fame or any other benefit in this world. Although the explanation and rationale of this unselfish work is only in Jnana Yoga, yet the natural divinity of man makes him love all sacrifice simply for the good of others, without any ulterior motive, whatever his creed or opinion. Again, with many the bondage of wealth is very great; and Karma Yoga is absolutely necessary for them as breaking the crystallisation that has gathered round their love of money.

Next is Bhakti Yoga. Bhakti or worship or love in some form or other is the easiest, pleasantest, and most natural way of man. The natural state of this universe is attraction; and that is surely followed by an ultimate disunion. Even so, love is the natural impetus of union in the human heart; and though itself a great cause of misery, properly directed towards the proper object, it brings deliverance. The object of Bhakti is God. Love cannot be without a subject and an object. The object of love again must be at first a being who can reciprocate our love. Therefore the God of love must be in some sense a human God. He must be a God of love. Aside from the question whether such a God exists or not, it is a fact that to those who have love in their heart this Absolute appears as a God of love, as personal.

The lower forms of worship, which embody the idea of God as a judge or punisher or someone to be obeyed through fear, do not deserve to be called love, although they are forms of worship gradually expanding into higher forms. We pass on to the consideration of love itself. We will illustrate love by a triangle, of which the first angle at the base is fearlessness. So long as there is fear, it is not love. Love banishes all fear. A mother with her baby will face a tiger to save her child. The second angle is that love never asks, never begs. The third or the apex is that love loves for the sake of love itself. Even the idea of object vanishes. Love is the only form in which love is loved. This is the highest abstraction and the same as the Absolute.

Next is Raja Yoga. This Yoga fits in with every one of these Yogas. It fits inquirers of all classes with or without any belief, and it is the real instrument of religious inquiry. As each science has its particular method of investigation, so is this Raja Yoga the method of religion. This science also is variously applied according to various constitutions. The chief parts are the Prânâyâma, concentration, and meditation. For those who believe in God, a symbolical name, such as Om or other sacred words received from a Guru, will be very helpful. Om is the greatest, meaning the Absolute. Meditating on the meaning of these holy names while repeating them is the chief practice.

Next is Jnana Yoga. This is divided into three parts. First: hearing the truth — that the Atman is the only reality and that everything else is Mâyâ (relativity). Second: reasoning upon this philosophy from all points of view. Third: giving up all further argumentation and realising the truth. This realisation comes from (1) being certain that Brahman is real and everything else is unreal; (2) giving up all desire for enjoyment; (3) controlling the senses and the mind; (4) intense desire to be free. Meditating on this reality always and reminding the soul of its real nature are the only ways in this Yoga. It is the highest, but most difficult. Many persons get an intellectual grasp of it, but very few attain realisation.

❑

1

Prayer

स तन्मयो ह्यमृत ईशसंस्थो ज्ञः सर्वगो भुवनस्यास्य गोप्ता।

य ईशेऽस्य जगतो नित्यमेव नान्यो हेतुर्विद्यत ईशनाय॥

यो ब्रह्माणं विदधाति पूर्वं यो वै वेदांश्च प्रहिणोति तस्मै।

तं ह देवं आत्मबुद्धिप्रकाशं मुमुक्षुर्वै शरणमहं प्रपद्ये॥

"He is the Soul of the Universe; He is Immortal; His is the Rulership; He is the All-knowing, the All-pervading, the Protector of the Universe, the Eternal Ruler. None else is there efficient to govern the world eternally. He who at the beginning of creation projected Brahmâ (i.e. the universal consciousness), and who delivered the Vedas unto him — seeking liberation I go for refuge unto that effulgent One, whose light turns the understanding towards the Âtman."

—Shvetâshvatara-Upanishad, VI. 17-18.

Definition of Bhakti

Bhakti Yoga is a real, genuine search after the Lord, a search beginning, continuing, and ending in love. One single moment of the madness of extreme love to God brings us eternal freedom.

"Bhakti", says Nârada in his explanation of the Bhakti-aphorisms, "is intense love to God"; "When a man gets it, he loves all, hates none; he becomes satisfied for ever"; "This love cannot be reduced to any earthly benefit", because so long as worldly desires last, that kind of love does not come; "Bhakti is greater than karma, greater than Yoga, because these are intended for an object in view, while Bhakti is its own fruition, its own means and its own end."

Bhakti has been the one constant theme of our sages. Apart from the special writers on Bhakti, such as Shândilya or Narada, the great commentators on the Vyâsa-Sutras, evidently advocates of knowledge (Jnâna), have also something very suggestive to say about love. Even when the commentator is anxious to explain many, if not all, of the texts so as to make them import a sort of dry knowledge, the Sutras, in the chapter on worship especially, do not lend themselves to be easily manipulated in that fashion.

There is not really so much difference between knowledge (Jnana) and love (Bhakti) as people sometimes imagine. We shall see, as we go on, that in the end they converge and meet at the same point. So also is it with Râja-Yoga, which when pursued as a means to attain liberation, and not (as unfortunately it frequently becomes in the hands of charlatans and mystery-mongers) as an instrument to hoodwink the unwary, leads us also to the same goal.

The one great advantage of Bhakti is that it is the easiest and the most natural way to reach the great divine end in view; its great disadvantage is that in its lower forms it oftentimes degenerates into hideous fanaticism. The fanatical crew in Hinduism, or Mohammedanism, or Christianity, have always been almost exclusively recruited from these worshippers on the lower planes of Bhakti. That singleness of attachment (Nishthâ) to a loved object, without which no genuine love can grow, is very often also the cause of the denunciation of everything else. All the weak and undeveloped minds in every religion or country have only one way of loving their own ideal, i.e. by hating every other ideal. Herein is the explanation of why the same man who is so lovingly attached to his own ideal of God, so devoted to his own ideal of religion, becomes a howling fanatic as soon as he sees or hears anything of any other ideal. This kind of love is somewhat like the canine instinct of guarding the master's property from intrusion; only, the instinct of the dog is better than the reason of man, for the dog never mistakes its master for an enemy in whatever dress he may come before it. Again, the fanatic loses all power of judgment. Personal considerations are in his case of such absorbing interest that to him it is no question at all what a man says — whether it is right or wrong; but the one thing he is always particularly careful to know is who says it. The same man who is kind, good, honest, and loving to people of his own opinion, will not hesitate to do the vilest deeds when they are directed against persons beyond the pale of his own religious brotherhood.

But this danger exists only in that stage of Bhakti which is called the preparatory (Gauni). When Bhakti has become ripe and has passed into that form which is called the supreme (Parâ), no more is there any fear of these hideous manifestations of fanaticism; that soul which is overpowered by this higher form of Bhakti is too near the God of Love to become an instrument for the diffusion of hatred.

It is not given to all of us to be harmonious in the building up of our characters in this life: yet we know that that character is of the noblest type in which all these three — knowledge and love and Yoga — are harmoniously fused. Three things are necessary for a bird to fly — the two wings and the tail as a rudder for steering. Jnana (Knowledge) is the one wing, Bhakti (Love) is the other, and Yoga is the tail that keeps up the balance. For those who cannot pursue all these three forms of worship together in harmony and take up, therefore, Bhakti alone as their way, it is necessary always to remember that forms and ceremonials, though absolutely necessary for the progressive soul, have no other value than taking us on to that state in which we feel the most intense love to God.

There is a little difference in opinion between the teachers of knowledge and those of love, though both admit the power of Bhakti. The Jnanis hold Bhakti to be an instrument of liberation, the Bhaktas look upon it both as the instrument and the thing to be attained. To my mind this is a distinction without much difference. In fact, Bhakti, when used as an instrument, really means a lower form of worship, and the higher form becomes inseparable from the lower form of realisation at a later stage. Each seems to lay a great stress upon his own peculiar method of worship, forgetting that with perfect love true knowledge is bound to come even unsought, and that from perfect knowledge true love is inseparable.

Bearing this in mind let us try to understand what the great Vedantic commentators have to say on the subject. In explaining the Sutra Âvrittirasakridupadeshât1, Bhagavân Shankara says, "Thus people say, 'He is devoted to the king, he is devoted to the Guru'; they say this of him who follows his Guru, and does so, having that following as the one end in view. Similarly they say, 'The loving wife meditates on her loving husband'; here also a kind of eager and continuous remembrance is meant." This is devotion according to Shankara.

"Meditation again is a constant remembrance (of the thing meditated upon) flowing like an unbroken stream of oil poured out from one vessel to another. When this kind of remembering has been attained (in relation to God) all bondages break. Thus it is spoken of in the scriptures regarding constant remembering as a means to liberation. This remembering again is of the same form as seeing, because it is of the same meaning as in the passage, 'When He who is far and near is seen, the bonds of the heart are broken, all doubts vanish, and all effects of work disappear' He who is near can be seen, but he who is far can only be remembered. Nevertheless the scripture says that he have to see Him who is near as well as Him who, is far, thereby indicating to us that the above kind of remembering is as good as seeing. This remembrance when exalted assumes the same form as seeing. . . . Worship is constant remembering as may be seen from the essential texts of scriptures. Knowing, which is the same as repeated worship, has been described as constant remembering. . . . Thus the memory, which has attained to the height of what is as good as direct perception, is spoken of in the Shruti as a means of liberation. 'This Atman is not to be reached through various sciences, nor by intellect, nor by much study of the Vedas. Whomsoever this Atman desires, by him is the Atman attained, unto him this Atman discovers Himself.' Here, after saying that mere hearing, thinking and meditating are not the means of attaining this Atman, it is said, 'Whom this Atman desires, by him the Atman is attained.' The extremely beloved is desired; by whomsoever this Atman is extremely beloved, he becomes the most beloved of the Atman. So that this beloved may attain the Atman, the Lord Himself helps. For it has been said by the Lord: 'Those who are constantly attached to Me and worship Me with love – I give that direction to their will by which they come to Me.' Therefore it is said that, to whomsoever this remembering, which is of the same form as direct perception, is very dear, because it is dear to the Object of such memory perception, he is desired by the Supreme Atman, by him the Supreme Atman is attained. This constant remembrance is denoted by the word Bhakti." So says Bhagavân Râmânuja in his commentary on the Sutra Athâto Brahma-jijnâsâ2.

In commenting on the Sutra of Patanjali, Ishvara pranidhânâdvâ, i.e. "Or by the worship of the Supreme Lord" – Bhoja says, "Pranidhâna is that sort of Bhakti in which, without seeking results, such as sense-enjoyments etc., all works are dedicated to that Teacher of teachers." Bhagavan Vyâsa also, when commenting on the same, defines Pranidhana as "the form of Bhakti by which the mercy of the Supreme Lord comes to the Yogi, and blesses him by granting him his desires". According to Shândilya, "Bhakti is intense love to God." The best definition is, however, that given by the king of Bhaktas, Prahlâda:

या प्रीतिरविवेकानां विषयेष्वनपायिनी।
त्वामनुस्मरतः सा मे हृदयान्मापसर्पतु॥

"That deathless love which the ignorant have for the fleeting objects of the senses – as I keep meditating on Thee – may not that love slip away from my heart!" Love! For whom? For the Supreme Lord Ishvara. Love for any other being, however great cannot be Bhakti; for, as Ramanuja says in his Shri Bhâshya, quoting an ancient Âchârya, i.e. a great teacher:

आब्रह्मस्तम्बपर्यन्ताः जगदन्तर्व्यवस्थिताः।
प्राणिनः कर्मजनितसंसारवशवर्तिनः॥
यतस्ततो न ते ध्याने ध्यानिनामुपकारकाः।
अविद्यान्तर्गतास्सर्वे ते हि संसारगोचराः॥

"From Brahmâ to a clump of grass, all things that live in the world are slaves of birth and death caused by Karma; therefore they cannot be helpful as objects of meditation, because they are all in ignorance and subject to change." In commenting on the word Anurakti used by Shandilya, the commentator Svapneshvara says that it means Anu, after, and Rakti, attachment; i.e. the attachment which comes after the knowledge of the nature and glory of God; else a blind attachment to any one, e.g. to wife or children, would be Bhakti. We plainly see, therefore, that Bhakti is a series or succession of mental efforts at religious realisation beginning with ordinary worship and ending in a supreme intensity of love for Ishvara.

Notes

1. Meditation is necessary, that having been often enjoined.
2. Hence follows a dissertation on Brahman.

❑

2

The Philosophy of Ishvara

Who is Ishvara? Janmâdyasya yatah – "From whom is the birth, continuation, and dissolution of the universe," – He is Ishvara – "the Eternal, the Pure, the Ever-Free, the Almighty, the All-Knowing, the All-Merciful, the Teacher of all teachers"; and above all, Sa Ishvarah anirvachaniya-premasvarupah – "He the Lord is, of His own nature, inexpressible Love." These certainly are the definitions of a Personal God. Are there then two Gods – the "Not this, not this," the Sat-chit-ânanda, the Existence-Knowledge-Bliss of the philosopher, and this God of Love of the Bhakta? No, it is the same Sat-chit-ananda who is also the God of Love, the impersonal and personal in one. It has always to be understood that the Personal God worshipped by the Bhakta is not separate or different from the Brahman. All is Brahman, the One without a second; only the Brahman, as unity or absolute, is too much of an abstraction to be loved and worshipped; so the Bhakta chooses the relative aspect of Brahman, that is, Ishvara, the Supreme Ruler. To use a simile: Brahman is as the clay or substance out of which an infinite variety of articles are fashioned. As clay, they are all one; but form or manifestation differentiates them. Before every one of them was made, they all existed potentially in the clay, and, of course, they are identical substantially; but when formed, and so long as the form remains, they are separate and different; the clay-mouse can never become a clay-elephant, because, as manifestations, form alone makes them what they are, though as unformed clay they are all one. Ishvara is the highest manifestation of the Absolute Reality, or in other words, the highest possible reading of the Absolute by the human mind. Creation is eternal, and so also is Ishvara.

In the fourth Pâda of the fourth chapter of his Sutras, after stating the almost infinite power and knowledge which will come to the liberated soul after the attainment of Moksha, Vyâsa makes the remark, in an aphorism, that none, however, will get the power of creating, ruling, and dissolving the universe, because that belongs to God alone. In explaining the Sutra it is easy for the dualistic commentators to show how it is ever impossible for a subordinate soul, Jiva, to have the infinite power and total independence of God. The thorough dualistic commentator Madhvâchârya deals with this passage in his usual summary method by quoting a verse from the Varâha Purâna.

In explaining this aphorism the commentator Râmânuja says, "This doubt being raised, whether among the powers of the liberated souls is included that unique power of the Supreme One, that is, of creation etc. of the universe and even the Lordship of all, or whether, without that, the glory of the liberated consists only in the direct perception of the Supreme One, we get as an argument the following: It is reasonable that the liberated get the Lordship of the universe, because the scriptures say, 'He attains to extreme sameness with the Supreme One and all his desires are realised.' Now extreme sameness and realisation of all desires cannot be attained without the unique power of the Supreme Lord, namely, that of governing the universe. Therefore, to attain the realisation of all desires and the extreme sameness with the Supreme, we must all admit that the liberated get the power of ruling the whole universe. To this we reply, that the liberated get all the powers except that of ruling the universe. Ruling the universe is guiding the form and the life and the desires of all the sentient and the non-sentient beings. The liberated ones from whom all that veils His true nature has been removed, only enjoy the unobstructed perception of the Brahman, but do not possess the power of ruling the universe. This is proved from the scriptural text, "From whom all these things are born, by which all that are born live, unto whom they, departing, return – ask about it. That is Brahman.' If this quality of ruling the universe be a quality common even to the liberated then this text would not apply as a definition of Brahman defining Him through His rulership of the universe. The uncommon attributes alone define a thing; therefore in texts like – 'My beloved boy, alone, in the beginning there existed the One without a second. That saw and felt, "I will give birth to the many." That projected heat.' – 'Brahman indeed alone existed in the beginning. That One evolved. That projected a blessed form, the Kshatra. All these gods are Kshatras: Varuna, Soma, Rudra, Parjanya, Yama, Mrityu, Ishâna.' – 'Atman indeed existed alone in the beginning; nothing else vibrated; He thought of projecting the world; He projected the world after.' – 'Alone Nârâyana existed; neither Brahmâ, nor Ishana, nor the Dyâvâ-Prithivi, nor the stars, nor water, nor fire, nor Soma, nor the sun. He did not take pleasure alone. He after His meditation had one daughter, the ten organs, etc.' – and in others as,

'Who living in the earth is separate from the earth, who living in the Atman, etc.' — the Shrutis speak of the Supreme One as the subject of the work of ruling the universe. . . . Nor in these descriptions of the ruling of the universe is there any position for the liberated soul, by which such a soul may have the ruling of the universe ascribed to it."

In explaining the next Sutra, Râmânuja says, "If you say it is not so, because there are direct texts in the Vedas in evidence to the contrary, these texts refer to the glory of the liberated in the spheres of the subordinate deities." This also is an easy solution of the difficulty. Although the system of Ramanuja admits the unity of the total, within that totality of existence there are, according to him, eternal differences. Therefore, for all practical purposes, this system also being dualistic, it was easy for Ramanuja to keep the distinction between the personal soul and the Personal God very clear.

We shall now try to understand what the great representative of the Advaita School has to say on the point. We shall see how the Advaita system maintains all the hopes and aspirations of the dualist intact, and at the same time propounds its own solution of the problem in consonance with the high destiny of divine humanity. Those who aspire to retain their individual mind even after liberation and to remain distinct will have ample opportunity of realising their aspirations and enjoying the blessing of the qualified Brahman. These are they who have been spoken of in the Bhâgavata Purâna thus: "O king, such are the, glorious qualities of the Lord that the sages whose only pleasure is in the Self, and from whom all fetters have fallen off, even they love the Omnipresent with the love that is for love›s sake." These are they who are spoken of by the Sânkhyas as getting merged in nature in this cycle, so that, after attaining perfection, they may come out in the next as lords of world-systems. But none of these ever becomes equal to God (Ishvara). Those who attain to that state where there is neither creation, nor created, nor creator, where there is neither knower, nor knowable, nor knowledge, where there is neither I, nor thou, nor he, where there is neither subject, nor object, nor relation, "there, who is seen by whom?" — such persons have gone beyond everything to "where words cannot go nor mind", gone to that which the Shrutis declare as "Not this, not this"; but for those who cannot, or will not reach this state, there will inevitably remain the triune vision of the one undifferentiated Brahman as nature, soul, and the interpenetrating sustainer of both — Ishvara. So, when Prahlâda forgot himself, he found neither the universe nor its cause; all was to him one Infinite, undifferentiated by name and form; but as soon as he remembered that he was Prahlada, there was the universe before him and with it the Lord of the universe — "the Repository of an infinite number of blessed qualities". So it was with the blessed Gopis. So long as they had lost sense of their own personal identity and individuality, they were all Krishnas, and when they began again to think of Him as the One to be worshipped, then they were Gopis again, and immediately

तासामाविरभूच्छौरिः स्मयमानमुखाम्बुजः ।
पीताम्बरधरः स्त्रग्वी साखान्मन्मथमन्मथः ॥

(Bhagavata)

— "Unto them appeared Krishna with a smile on His lotus face, clad in yellow robes and having garlands on, the embodied conqueror (in beauty) of the god of love."

Now to go back to our Acharya Shankara: "Those", he says, "who by worshipping the qualified Brahman attain conjunction with the Supreme Ruler, preserving their own mind — is their glory limited or unlimited? This doubt arising, we get as an argument: Their glory should be unlimited because of the scriptural texts, 'They attain their own kingdom', 'To him all the gods offer worship', 'Their desires are fulfilled in all the worlds'. As an answer to this, Vyasa writes, 'Without the power of ruling the universe.' Barring the power of creation etc. of the universe, the other powers such as Animâ etc. are acquired by the liberated. As to ruling the universe, that belongs to the eternally perfect Ishvara. Why? Because He is the subject of all the scriptural texts as regards creation etc., and the liberated souls are not mentioned therein in any connection whatsoever. The Supreme Lord indeed is alone engaged in ruling the universe. The texts as to creation etc. all point to Him. Besides, there is given the adjective 'ever-perfect'. Also the scriptures say that the powers Anima etc. of the others are from the search after and the worship of God. Therefore they have no place in the ruling of the universe. Again, on account of their possessing their own minds, it is possible that their wills may differ, and that, whilst one desires creation, another may desire destruction. The only way of avoiding this conflict is to make all wills subordinate to some one will. Therefore the conclusion is that the wills of the liberated are dependent on the will of the Supreme Ruler."

Bhakti, then, can be directed towards Brahman, only in His personal aspect.

क्लेशोऽधिकतरस्तेषामव्यक्तासक्तचेतसाम्

– "The way is more difficult for those whose mind is attached to the Absolute!" Bhakti has to float on smoothly with the current of our nature. True it is that we cannot have; any idea of the Brahman which is not anthropomorphic, but is it not equally true of everything we know? The greatest psychologist the world has ever known, Bhagavan Kapila, demonstrated ages ago that human consciousness is one of the elements in the make-up of all the objects of our perception and conception, internal as well as external. Beginning with our bodies and going up to Ishvara, we may see that every object of our perception is this consciousness plus something else, whatever that may be; and this unavoidable mixture is what we ordinarily think of as reality. Indeed it is, and ever will be, all of the reality that is possible for the human mind to know. Therefore to say that Ishvara is unreal, because He is anthropomorphic, is sheer nonsense. It sounds very much like the occidentals squabble on idealism and realism, which fearful-looking quarrel has for its foundation a mere play on the word "real". The idea of Ishvara covers all the ground ever denoted and connoted by the word real, and Ishvara is as real as anything else in the universe; and after all, the word real means nothing more than what has now been pointed out. Such is our philosophical conception of Ishvara.

❑

3

Spiritual Realisation: The Aim of Bhakti Yoga

To the Bhakta these dry details are necessary only to strengthen his will; beyond that they are of no use to him. For he is treading on a path which is fitted very soon to lead him beyond the hazy and turbulent regions of reason, to lead him to the realm of realisation. He, soon, through the mercy of the Lord, reaches a plane where pedantic and powerless reason is left far behind, and the mere intellectual groping through the dark gives place to the daylight of direct perception. He no more reasons and believes, he almost perceives. He no more argues, he senses. And is not this seeing God, and feeling God, and enjoying God higher than everything else? Nay, Bhaktas have not been wanting who have maintained that it is higher than even Moksha – liberation. And is it not also the highest utility? There are people – and a good many of them too – in the world who are convinced that only that is of use and utility which brings to man creature-comforts. Even religion, God, eternity, soul, none of these is of any use to them, as they do not bring them money or physical comfort. To such, all those things which do not go to gratify the senses and appease the appetites are of no utility. In every mind, utility, however, is conditioned by its own peculiar wants. To men, therefore, who never rise higher than eating, drinking, begetting progeny, and dying, the only gain is in sense enjoyments; and they must wait and go through many more births and reincarnations to learn to feel even the faintest necessity for anything higher. But those to whom the eternal interests of the soul are of much higher value than the fleeting interests of this mundane life, to whom the gratification of the senses is but like the thoughtless play of the baby, to them God and the love of God form the highest and the only utility of human existence. Thank God there are some such still living in this world of too much worldliness.

Bhakti Yoga, as we have said, is divided into the Gauni or the preparatory, and the Parâ or the supreme forms. We shall find, as we go on, how in the preparatory stage we unavoidably stand in need of many concrete helps to enable us to get on; and indeed the mythological and symbological parts of all religions are natural growths which early environ the aspiring soul and help it Godward. It is also a significant fact that spiritual giants have been produced only in those systems of religion where there is an exuberant growth of rich mythology and ritualism. The dry fanatical forms of religion which attempt to eradicate all that is poetical, all that is beautiful and sublime, all that gives a firm grasp to the infant mind tottering in its Godward way — the forms which attempt to break down the very ridge-poles of the spiritual roof, and in their ignorant and superstitious conceptions of truth try to drive away all that is life-giving, all that furnishes the formative material to the spiritual plant growing in the human soul — such forms of religion too soon find that all that is left to them is but an empty shell, a contentless frame of words and sophistry with perhaps a little flavour of a kind of social scavengering or the so-called spirit of reform.

The vast mass of those whose religion is like this, are conscious or unconscious materialists — the end and aim of their lives here and hereafter being enjoyment, which indeed is to them the alpha and the omega of human life, and which is their Ishtâpurta; work like street-cleaning and scavengering, intended for the material comfort of man is, according to them, the be-all and end-all of human existence; and the sooner the followers of this curious mixture of ignorance and fanaticism come out in their true colours and join, as they well deserve to do, the ranks of atheists and materialists, the better will it be for the world. One ounce of the practice of righteousness and of spiritual Self-realisation outweighs tons and tons of frothy talk and nonsensical sentiments. Show us one, but one gigantic spiritual genius growing out of all this dry dust of ignorance and fanaticism; and if you cannot, close your mouths, open the windows of your hearts to the clear light of truth, and sit like children at the feet of those who know what they are talking about — the sages of India. Let us then listen attentively to what they say.

❑

4

The Need of Guru

Every soul is destined to be perfect, and every being, in the end, will attain the state of perfection. Whatever we are now is the result of our acts and thoughts in the past; and whatever we shall be in the future will be the result of what we think and do now. But this, the shaping of our own destinies, does not preclude our receiving help from outside; nay, in the vast majority of cases such help is absolutely necessary. When it comes, the higher powers and possibilities of the soul are quickened, spiritual life is awakened, growth is animated, and man becomes holy and perfect in the end.

This quickening impulse cannot be derived from books. The soul can only receive impulses from another soul, and from nothing else. We may study books all our lives, we may become very intellectual, but in the end we find that we have not developed at all spiritually. It is not true that a high order of intellectual development always goes hand in hand with a proportionate development of the spiritual side in Man. In studying books we are sometimes deluded into thinking that thereby we are being spiritually helped; but if we analyse the effect of the study of books on ourselves, we shall find that at the utmost it is only our intellect that derives profit from such studies, and not our inner spirit. This inadequacy of books to quicken spiritual growth is the reason why, although almost every one of us can speak most wonderfully on spiritual matters, when it comes to action and the living of a truly spiritual life, we find ourselves so awfully deficient. To quicken the spirit, the impulse must come from another soul.

The person from whose soul such impulse comes is called the Guru – the teacher; and the person to whose soul the impulse is conveyed is called the Shishya – the student. To convey such an impulse to any soul, in the first place, the soul from which it proceeds must possess the power of transmitting it, as it were, to another; and in the second place, the soul to which it is transmitted must be fit to receive it. The seed must be a living seed, and the field must be ready ploughed; and when both these conditions are fulfilled, a wonderful growth of genuine religion takes place.

"The true preacher of religion has to be of wonderful capabilities, and clever shall his hearer be" –

आश्चर्यो वक्ता कुशलोऽस्य लब्धा;

and when both of these are really wonderful and extraordinary, then will a splendid spiritual awakening result, and not otherwise. Such alone are the real teachers, and such alone are also the real students, the real aspirants. All others are only playing with spirituality. They have just a little curiosity awakened, just a little intellectual aspiration kindled in them, but are merely standing on the outward fringe of the horizon of religion. There is no doubt some value even in that, as it may in course of time result in the awakening of a real thirst for religion; and it is a mysterious law of nature that as soon as the field is ready, the seed must and does come; as soon as the soul earnestly desires to have religion, the transmitter of the religious force must and does appear to help that soul. When the power that attracts the light of religion in the receiving soul is full and strong, the power which answers to that attraction and sends in light does come as a matter of course.

There are, however, certain great dangers in the way. There is, for instance, the danger to the receiving soul of its mistaking momentary emotions for real religious yearning. We may study that in ourselves. Many a time in our lives, somebody dies whom we loved; we receive a blow; we feel that the world is slipping between our fingers, that we want something surer and higher, and that we must become religious. In a few days that wave of feeling has passed away, and we are left stranded just where we were before. We are all of us often mistaking such impulses for real thirst after religion; but as long as these momentary emotions are thus mistaken, that continuous, real craving of the soul for religion will not come, and we shall not find the true transmitter of spirituality into our nature. So whenever we are tempted to complain of our search after the truth that we desire so much, proving vain, instead of so complaining, our first duty ought to be to look into our own souls and find whether the craving in the heart is real. Then in the vast majority of cases it would be discovered that we were not fit for receiving the truth, that there was no real thirst for spirituality.

There are still greater dangers in regard to the transmitter, the Guru. There are many who, though immersed in ignorance, yet, in the pride of their hearts, fancy they know everything, and not only do not stop there, but offer to take others on their shoulders; and thus the blind leading the blind, both fall into the ditch.

अविद्यायामन्तरे वर्तमानाः स्वयं धीराः पण्डितम्मन्यमानाः ।

दन्द्रम्यमाणाः परियन्ति मूढा अन्धेनैव नीयमाना यथान्धाः ॥

— "Fools dwelling in darkness, wise in their own conceit, and puffed up with vain knowledge, go round and round staggering to and fro, like blind men led by the blind." — (Katha Up., I. ii. 5). The world is full of these. Every one wants to be a teacher, every beggar wants to make a gift of a million dollars! Just as these beggars are ridiculous, so are these teachers.

❑

5

Qualifications of The Aspirant and The Teacher

How are we to know a teacher, then? The sun requires no torch to make him visible, we need not light a candle in order to see him. When the sun rises, we instinctively become aware of the fact, and when a teacher of men comes to help us, the soul will instinctively know that truth has already begun to shine upon it. Truth stands on its own evidence, it does not require any other testimony to prove it true, it is self effulgent. It penetrates into the innermost corners of our nature, and in its presence the whole universe stands up and says, "This is truth." The teachers whose wisdom and truth shine like the light of the sun are the very greatest the world has known, and they are worshipped as God by the major portion of mankind. But we may get help from comparatively lesser ones also; only we ourselves do not possess intuition enough to judge properly of the man from whom we receive teaching and guidance; so there ought to be certain tests, certain conditions, for the teacher to satisfy, as there are also for the taught.

The conditions necessary for the taught are purity, a real thirst after knowledge, and perseverance. No impure soul can be really religious. Purity in thought, speech, and act is absolutely necessary for any one to be religious. As to the thirst after knowledge, it is an old law that we all get whatever we want. None of us can get anything other than what we fix our hearts upon. To pant for religion truly is a very difficult thing, not at all so easy as we generally imagine. Hearing religious talks or reading religious books is no proof yet of a real want felt in the heart; there must be a continuous struggle, a constant fight, an unremitting grappling with our lower nature, till the higher want is actually felt and the victory is achieved. It is not a question of one or two days, of years, or of lives; the struggle may have to go on for hundreds of lifetimes. The success sometimes may come immediately, but we must be ready to wait patiently even for what may look like an infinite length of time. The student who sets out with such a spirit of perseverance will surely find success and realisation at last.

In regard to the teacher, we must see that he knows the spirit of the scriptures. The whole world reads Bibles, Vedas, and Korans; but they are all only words, syntax, etymology, philology, the dry bones of religion. The teacher who deals too much in words and allows the mind to be carried away by the force of words loses the spirit. It is the knowledge of the spirit of the scriptures alone that constitutes the true religious teacher. The network of the words of the scriptures is like a huge forest in which the human mind often loses itself and finds no way out.

शब्दजालं महारण्यं चित्तभ्रमणकारणम्।

— "The network of words is a big forest; it is the cause of a curious wandering of the mind." "The various methods of joining words, the various methods of speaking in beautiful language, the various methods of explaining the diction of the scriptures are only for the disputations and enjoyment of the learned, they do not conduce to the development of spiritual perception"

वाग्वैखरी शब्दझरी शास्त्रव्याख्यानकौशलम्।

वैदुष्यं विदुषां तद्वद् भुक्तये न तु मुक्तये॥

— Those who employ such methods to impart religion to others are only desirous to show off their learning, so that the world may praise them as great scholars. You will find that no one of the great teachers of the world ever went into these various explanations of the text; there is with them no attempt at "text-torturing", no eternal playing upon the meaning of words and their roots. Yet they nobly taught, while others who have nothing to teach have taken up a word sometimes and written a three-volume book on its origin, on the man who used it first, and on what that man was accustomed to eat, and how long he slept, and so on.

Bhagavân Ramakrishna used to tell a story of some men who went into a mango orchard and busied themselves in counting the leaves, the twigs, and the branches, examining their colour, comparing their size, and noting down everything most carefully, and then got up a learned discussion on each of these topics, which were undoubtedly highly interesting to them. But one of them, more sensible than the others, did not care for all these things. and instead thereof, began to eat the mango fruit. And was he not wise? So leave this counting of leaves and twigs and note-taking to others. This kind of work has its proper place, but not here in the spiritual domain. You never see a strong spiritual man among these "leaf counters". Religion, the highest aim, the highest glory of man, does not require so much labour. If you want to be a Bhakta, it is not at all necessary for you to know whether Krishna was born in Mathurâ or in Vraja, what he was doing, or just the exact date on which he pronounced the teachings of the Gitâ. You only require to feel the craving for the beautiful lessons of duty and love in the Gita. All the other particulars about it and its author are for the enjoyment of the learned. Let them have what they desire. Say "Shântih, Shântih" to their learned controversies, and let us "eat the mangoes".

The second condition necessary in the teacher is — sinlessness. The question is often asked, "Why should we look into the character and personality of a teacher? We have only to judge of what he says, and take that up." This is not right. If a man wants to teach me something of dynamics, or chemistry, or any other physical science, he may be anything he likes, because what the physical sciences require is merely an intellectual equipment; but in the spiritual sciences it is impossible from first to last that there can be any spiritual light in the soul that is impure. What religion can an impure man teach? The sine qua non of acquiring spiritual truth for one›s self or for imparting it to others is the purity of heart and soul. A vision of God or a glimpse of the beyond never comes until the soul is pure. Hence with the teacher of religion we must see first what he is, and then what he says. He must be perfectly pure, and then alone comes the value of his words, because he is only then the true "transmitter". What can he transmit if he has not spiritual power in himself? There must be the worthy vibration of spirituality in the mind of the teacher, so that it may be sympathetically conveyed to the mind of the taught. The function of the teacher is indeed an affair of the transference of something, and not one of mere stimulation of the existing intellectual or other faculties in the taught. Something real and appreciable as an influence comes from the teacher and goes to the taught. Therefore the teacher must be pure.

The third condition is in regard to the motile. The teacher must not teach with any ulterior selfish motive — for money, name, or fame; his work must be simply out of love, out of pure love for mankind at large. The only medium through which spiritual force can be transmitted is love. Any selfish motive, such as the desire for gain or for name, will immediately destroy this conveying median. God is love, and only he who has known God as love can be a teacher of godliness and God to man.

When you see that in your teacher these conditions are all fulfilled, you are safe; if they are not, it is unsafe to allow yourself to be taught by him, for there is the great danger that, if he cannot convey goodness to your heart, he may convey wickedness. This danger must by all means be guarded against.

श्रोत्रियोऽवृजिनोऽकामहतो यो ब्रह्मवित्तम:

— "He who is learned in the scriptures, sinless, unpolluted by lust, and is the greatest knower of the Brahman" is the real teacher.

From what has been said, it naturally follows that we cannot be taught to love, appreciate, and assimilate religion everywhere and by everybody. The "books in the running brooks, sermons in stones, and good in everything" is all very true as a poetical figure: but nothing can impart to a man a single grain of truth unless he has the undeveloped germs of it in himself. To whom do the stones and brooks preach sermons? To the human soul, the lotus of whose inner holy shrine is already quick with life. And the light which causes the beautiful opening out of this lotus comes always from the good and wise teacher. When the heart has thus been opened, it becomes fit to receive teaching from the stones or the brooks, the stars, or the sun, or the moon, or from any thing which has its existence in our divine universe; but the unopened heart will see in them nothing but mere stones or mere brooks. A blind man may go to a museum, but he will not profit by it in any way; his eyes must be opened first, and then alone he will be able to learn what the things in the museum can teach.

This eye-opener of the aspirant after religion is the teacher. With the teacher, therefore, our relationship is the same as that between an ancestor and his descendant. Without faith, humility, submission, and veneration in our hearts towards our religious teacher, there cannot be any growth of religion in us; and it is a significant fact that, where this kind of relation between the teacher and the taught prevails, there alone gigantic spiritual men are growing; while in those countries which have neglected to keep up this kind of relation the religious teacher has become a mere lecturer, the teacher expecting his five dollars and the person taught expecting his brain to be filled with the teacher's words, and each going his own way after this much has been done. Under such circumstances spirituality becomes almost an unknown quantity. There is none to transmit it and none to have it transmitted to. Religion with such people becomes business; they think they can obtain it with their dollars. Would to God that religion could be obtained so easily! But unfortunately it cannot be.

Religion, which is the highest knowledge and the highest wisdom, cannot be bought, nor can it be acquired from books. You may thrust your head into all the corners of the world, you may explore the Himalayas, the Alps, and the

Caucasus, you may sound the bottom of the sea and pry into every nook of Tibet and the desert of Gobi, you will not find it anywhere until your heart is ready for receiving it and your teacher has come. And when that divinely appointed teacher comes, serve him with childlike confidence and simplicity, freely open your heart to his influence, and see in him God manifested. Those who come to seek truth with such a spirit of love and veneration, to them the Lord of Truth reveals the most wonderful things regarding truth, goodness, and beauty.

❑

6

Incarnate Teachers and Incarnation

Wherever His name is spoken, that very place is holy. How much more so is the man who speaks His name, and with what veneration ought we to approach that man out of whom comes to us spiritual truth! Such great teachers of spiritual truth are indeed very few in number in this world, but the world is never altogether without them. They are always the fairest flowers of human life –

अहेतुकदयासिन्धुः

– "the ocean of mercy without any motive".

आचार्यं मां विजानीयात्

– "Know the Guru to be Me", says Shri Krishna in the Bhagavata.

The moment the world is absolutely bereft of these, it becomes a hideous hell and hastens on to its destruction.

Higher and nobler than all ordinary ones are another set of teachers, the Avatâras of Ishvara, in the world. They can transmit spirituality with a touch, even with a mere wish. The lowest and the most degraded characters become in one second saints at their command. They are the Teachers of all teachers, the highest manifestations of God through man. We cannot see God except through them. We cannot help worshipping them; and indeed they are the only ones whom we are bound to worship.

No man can really see God except through these human manifestations. If we try to see God otherwise, we make for ourselves a hideous caricature of Him and believe the caricature to be no worse than the original. There is a story of an ignorant man who was asked to make an image of the God Shiva, and who, after days of hard struggle, manufactured only the image of a monkey. So whenever we try to think of God as He is in His absolute perfection, we invariably meet with the most miserable failure, because as long as we are men, we cannot conceive Him as anything higher than man. The time will come when we shall transcend our human nature and know Him as He is; but as long as we are men, we must worship Him in man and as man. Talk as you may, try as you may, you cannot think of God except as a man. You may deliver great intellectual discourses on God and on all things under the sun, become great rationalists and prove to your satisfaction that all these accounts of the Avataras of God as man are nonsense. But let us come for a moment to practical common sense. What is there behind this kind of remarkable intellect? Zero, nothing, simply so much froth. When next you hear a man delivering a great intellectual lecture against this worship of the Avataras of God, get hold of him and ask what his idea of God is, what he understands by "omnipotence", "omnipresence", and all similar terms, beyond the spelling of the words. He really means nothing by them; he cannot formulate as their meaning any idea unaffected by his own human nature; he is no better off in this matter than the man in the street who has not read a single book. That man in the street, however, is quiet and does not disturb the peace of the world, while this big talker creates disturbance and misery among mankind. Religion is, after all, realisation, and we must make the sharpest distinction between talk; and intuitive experience. What we experience in the depths of our souls is realisation. Nothing indeed is so uncommon as common sense in regard to this matter.

By our present constitution we are limited and bound to see God as man. If, for instance the buffaloes want to worship God, they will, in keeping with their own nature, see Him as a huge buffalo; if a fish wants to worship God, it will have to form an Idea of Him as a big fish, and man has to think of Him as man. And these various conceptions are not due to morbidly active imagination. Man, the buffalo, and the fish all may be supposed to represent so many different vessels, so to say. All these vessels go to the sea of God to get filled with water, each according to its own shape and capacity; in the man the water takes the shape of man, in the buffalo, the shape of a buffalo and in the fish, the shape of a fish. In each of these vessels there is the same water of the sea of God. When men see Him, they see Him as man, and the animals, if they have any conception of God at all, must see Him as animal each according to its own ideal. So we cannot help seeing God as man, and, therefore, we are bound to worship Him as man. There is no other way.

Two kinds of men do not worship God as man — the human brute who has no religion, and the Paramahamsa who has risen beyond all the weaknesses of humanity and has transcended the limits of his own human nature. To him all nature has become his own Self. He alone can worship God as He is. Here, too, as in all other cases, the two extremes meet. The extreme of ignorance and the other extreme of knowledge — neither of these go through acts of worship. The human brute does not worship because of his ignorance, and the Jivanmuktas (free souls) do not worship because they have realised God in themselves. Being between these two poles of existence, if any one tells you that he is not going to worship God as man, take kindly care of that man; he is, not to use any harsher term, an irresponsible talker; his religion is for unsound and empty brains.

God understands human failings and becomes man to do good to humanity:

यदा यदा हि धर्मस्य ग्लानिर्भवति भारत।
अभ्युत्थानमधर्मस्य तदात्मानं सृजाम्यहम्॥
परित्राणाय साधूनां विनाशाय च दुष्कृताम्।
धर्मसंस्थापनार्थाय सम्भवामि युगे युगे॥

— "Whenever virtue subsides and wickedness prevails, I manifest Myself. To establish virtue, to destroy evil, to save the good I come from Yuga (age) to Yuga."

अवजानन्ति मां मूढा मानुषीं तनुमाश्रितम्।
परं भावमजानन्तो मम भूतमहेश्वरम्॥

— "Fools deride Me who have assumed the human form, without knowing My real nature as the Lord of the universe." Such is Shri Krishna's declaration in the Gita on Incarnation. "When a huge tidal wave comes," says Bhagavan Shri Ramakrishna, "all the little brooks and ditches become full to the brim without any effort or consciousness on their own part; so when an Incarnation comes, a tidal wave of spirituality breaks upon the world, and people feel spirituality almost full in the air."

❑

7

The Mantra - Om: Word and Wisdom

But we are now considering not these Mahâ-purushas, the great Incarnations, but only the Siddha-Gurus (teachers who have attained the goal); they, as a rule, have to convey the gems of spiritual wisdom to the disciple by means of words (Mantras) to be meditated upon. What are these Mantras? The whole of this universe has, according to Indian philosophy, both name and form (Nâma-Rupa) as its conditions of manifestation. In the human microcosm, there cannot be a single wave in the mind-stuff (Chittavritti) unconditioned by name and form. If it be true that nature is built throughout on the same plan, this kind of conditioning by name and form must also be the plan of the building of the whole of the cosmos.

यथा एकेन मृत्पिण्डेन सर्वं मृन्मयं विज्ञातं स्यात्

– "As one lump of clay being known, all things of clay are known", so the knowledge of the microcosm must lead to the knowledge of the macrocosm. Now form is the outer crust, of which the name or the idea is the inner essence or kernel. The body is the form, and the mind or the Antahkarana is the name, and sound-symbols are universally associated with Nâma (name) in all beings having the power of speech. In the individual man the thought-waves rising in the limited Mahat or Chitta (mind-stuff), must manifest themselves, first as words, and then as the more concrete forms.

In the universe, Brahmâ or Hiranyagarbha or the cosmic Mahat first manifested himself as name, and then as form, i.e. as this universe. All this expressed sensible universe is the form, behind which stands the eternal inexpressible Sphota, the manifester as Logos or Word. This eternal Sphota, the essential eternal material of all ideas or names is the power through which the Lord creates the universe, nay, the Lord first becomes conditioned as the Sphota, and then evolves Himself out as the yet more concrete sensible universe.

This Sphota has one word as its only possible symbol, and this is the ओं (Om).

And as by no possible means of analysis can we separate the word from the idea this Om and the eternal Sphota are inseparable; and therefore, it is out of this holiest of all holy words, the mother of all names and forms, the eternal Om, that the whole universe may be supposed to have been created. But it may be said that, although thought and word are inseparable, yet as there may be various word-symbols for the same thought, it is not necessary that this particular word Om should be the word representative of the thought, out of which the universe has become manifested. To this objection we reply that this Om is the only possible symbol which covers the whole ground, and there is none other like it. The Sphota is the material of all words, yet it is not any definite word in its fully formed state. That is to say, if all the peculiarities which distinguish one word from another be removed, then what remains will be the Sphota; therefore this Sphota is called the Nâda-Brahma, the Sound-Brahman.

Now, as every word-symbol, intended to express the inexpressible Sphota, will so particularise it that it will no longer be the Sphota, that symbol which particularises it the least and at the same time most approximately expresses its nature, will be the truest symbol thereof; and this is the Om, and the Om only;

> because these three letters अ उ म (A.U.M.), pronounced incombination as Om, may well be the generalised symbol of all possible sounds. The letter A is the least differentiated of all sounds, therefore Krishna says in the Gita अक्षराणां अकारोऽस्मि — "I am A among the letters".

Again, all articulate sounds are produced in the space within the mouth beginning with the root of the tongue and ending in the lips — the throat sound is A, and M is the last lip sound, and the U exactly represents the rolling forward of the impulse which begins at the root of the tongue till it ends in the lips. If properly pronounced, this Om will represent the whole phenomenon of sound-production, and no other word can do this; and this, therefore, is the fittest symbol of the Sphota, which is the real meaning of the Om. And as the symbol can never be separated from the thing signified, the Om and the Sphota are one. And as the Sphota, being the finer side of the manifested universe, is nearer to God and is indeed that first manifestation of divine wisdom this Om is truly symbolic of God. Again, just as the "One only" Brahman, the Akhanda-Sachchidânanda, the undivided Existence-Knowledge-Bliss, can be conceived by imperfect human souls only from particular standpoints and associated with particular qualities, so this universe, His body, has also to be thought of along the line of the thinker's mind.

This direction of the worshipper's mind is guided by its prevailing elements or Tattvas. The result is that the same God will be seen in various manifestations as the possessor of various predominant qualities, and the same universe will appear as full of manifold forms. Even as in the case of the least differentiated and the most universal symbol Om, thought and sound-symbol are seen to be inseparably associated with each other, so also this law of their inseparable association applies to the many differentiated views of God and the universe: each of them therefore must have a particular word-symbol to express it. These word-symbols, evolved out of the deepest spiritual perception of sages, symbolise and express, as nearly as possible the particular view of God and the universe they stand for. And as the Om represents the Akhanda, the undifferentiated Brahman, the others represent the Khanda or the differentiated views of the same Being; and they are all helpful to divine meditation and the acquisition of true knowledge.

❑

8

Worship of Substitutes and Images

The next points to be considered are the worship of Pratikas or of things more or less satisfactory as substitutes for God, and the worship of Pratimâs or images. What is the worship of God through a Pratika?

It is अब्रह्मणि ब्रह्मदृष्ट्यऽनुसन्धानम्

— Joining the mind with devotion to that which is not Brahman, taking it to be Brahman" — says Bhagavân Râmânuja. "Worship the mind as Brahman this is internal; and the Âkâsha as Brahman, this is with regard to the Devas", says Shankara. The mind is an internal Pratika, the Akasha is an external one, and both have to be worshipped as substitutes of God. He continues, "Similarly — 'the Sun is Brahman, this is the command', 'He who worships Name as Brahman' — in all such passages the doubt arises as to the worship of Pratikas." The word Pratika means going towards; and worshipping a Pratika is worshipping something as a substitute which is, in some one or more respects, like Brahman more and more, but is not Brahman. Along with the Pratikas mentioned in the Shrutis there are various others to be found in the Purânas and the Tantras. In this kind of Pratika-worship may be included all the various forms of Pitri-worship and Deva-worship.

Now worshipping Ishvara and Him alone is Bhakti; the worship of anything else — Deva, or Pitri, or any other being — cannot be Bhakti. The various kinds of worship of the various Devas are all to be included in ritualistic Karma, which gives to the worshipper only a particular result in the form of some celestial enjoyment, but can neither give rise to Bhakti nor lead to Mukti. One thing, therefore, has to be carefully borne in mind. If, as it may happen in some cases, the highly philosophic ideal, the supreme Brahman, is dragged down by Pratika-worship to the level of the Pratika, and the Pratika itself is taken to be the Atman of the worshipper or his Antaryâmin (Inner Ruler), the worshipper gets entirely misled, as no Pratika can really be the Atman of the worshipper.

But where Brahman Himself is the object of worship, and the Pratika stands only as a substitute or a suggestion thereof, that is to say, where, through the Pratika the omnipresent Brahman is worshipped — the Pratika itself being idealised into the cause of all, Brahman — the worship is positively beneficial; nay, it is absolutely necessary for all mankind until they have all got beyond the primary or preparatory state of the mind in regard to worship. When, therefore, any gods or other beings are worshipped in and for themselves, such worship is only a ritualistic Karma; and as a Vidyâ (science) it gives us only the fruit belonging to that particular Vidya; but when the Devas or any other beings are looked upon as Brahman and worshipped, the result obtained is the same as by the worshipping of Ishvara. This explains how, in many cases, both in the Shrutis and the Smritis, a god, or a sage, or some other extraordinary being is taken up and lifted, as it were, out of his own nature and idealised into Brahman, and is then worshipped. Says the Advaitin, "Is not everything Brahman when the name and the form have been removed from it?" "Is not He, the Lord, the innermost Self of every one?" says the Vishishtâdvaitin.

फलम् आदित्याद्युपासनेषु ब्रह्मैव दास्यति सर्वाध्यक्षत्वात्

— "The fruition of even the worship of Adityas etc. Brahman Himself bestows, because He is the Ruler of all." Says Shankara in his Brahma-Sutra-Bhâsya—

ईदृशं चात्र ब्रह्मण उपास्यत्वं यतः प्रतीकेषु
तत्दृष्ट्याध्यारोपणं प्रतिमादिषु इव विष्णवादीनाम्।

"Here in this way does Brahman become the object of worship, because He, as Brahman, is superimposed on the Pratikas, just as Vishnu etc. are superimposed upon images etc."

The same ideas apply to the worship of the Pratimas as to that of the Pratikas; that is to say, if the image stands for a god or a saint, the worship is not the result of Bhakti, and does not lead lo liberation; but if it stands for the one God, the worship thereof will bring both Bhakti and Mukti. Of the principal religions of the world we see Vedantism, Buddhism, and certain forms of Christianity freely using images; only two religions, Mohammedanism and Protestantism, refuse such help. Yet the Mohammedans use the grave of their saints and martyrs almost in the place of images; and the Protestants, in rejecting all concrete helps to religion, are drifting away every year farther and farther from spirituality till at present there is scarcely any difference between the advanced Protestants and the followers of August Comte, or agnostics who preach ethics alone. Again, in Christianity and Mohammedanism whatever exists of image worship is made to fall under that category in which the Pratika or the Pratima is worshipped in itself, but not as a "help to the vision" (Drishtisaukaryam) of God; therefore it is at best only of the nature of ritualistic Karmas and cannot produce either Bhakti or Mukti. In this form of image-worship, the allegiance of the soul is given to other things than Ishvara, and, therefore, such use of images, or graves, or temples, or tombs, is real idolatry; it is in itself neither sinful nor wicked – it is a rite – a Karma, and worshippers must and will get the fruit thereof.

❑

9

The Chosen Ideal

The next thing to be considered is what we know as Ishta-Nishthâ. One who aspires to be a Bhakta must know that "so many opinions are so many ways". He must know that all the various sects of the various religions are the various manifestations of the glory of the same Lord. "They call You by so many names; they divide You, as it were, by different names, yet in each one of these is to be found Your omnipotence....You reach the worshipper through all of these, neither is there any special time so long as the soul has intense love for You. You are so easy of approach; it is my misfortune that I cannot love You." Not only this, the Bhakta must take care not to hate, nor even to criticise those radiant sons of light who are the founders of various sects; he must not even hear them spoken ill of. Very few indeed are those who are at once the possessors of an extensive sympathy and power of appreciation, as well as an intensity of love. We find, as a rule, that liberal and sympathetic sects lose the intensity of religious feeling, and in their hands, religion is apt to degenerate into a kind of politico-social club life. On the other hand, intensely narrow sectaries, whilst displaying a very commendable love of their own ideals, are seen to have acquired every particle of that love by hating every one who is not of exactly the same opinions as themselves. Would to God that this world was full of men who were as intense in their love as worldwide in their sympathies! But such are only few and far between. Yet we know that it is practicable to educate large numbers of human beings into the ideal of a wonderful blending of both the width and the intensity of love; and the way to do that is by this path of the Istha-Nishtha or "steadfast devotion to the chosen ideal". Every sect of every religion presents only one ideal of its own to mankind, but the eternal Vedantic religion opens to mankind an infinite number of doors for ingress into the inner shrine of divinity, and places before humanity an almost inexhaustible array of ideals, there being in each of them a manifestation of the Eternal One. With the kindest solicitude, the Vedanta points out to aspiring men and women the numerous roads, hewn out of the solid rock of the realities of human life, by the glorious sons, or human manifestations, of God, in the past and in the present, and stands with outstretched arms to welcome all — to welcome even those that are yet to be — to that Home of Truth and that Ocean of Bliss, wherein the human soul, liberated from the net of Mâyâ, may transport itself with perfect freedom and with eternal joy.

Bhakti Yoga, therefore, lays on us the imperative command not to hate or deny any one of the various paths that lead to salvation. Yet the growing plant must be hedged round to protect it until it has grown into a tree. The tender plant of spirituality will die if exposed too early to the action of a constant change of ideas and ideals. Many people, in the name of what may be called religious liberalism, may be seen feeding their idle curiosity with a continuous succession of different ideals. With them, hearing new things grows into a kind of disease, a sort of religious drink-mania. They want to hear new things just by way of getting a temporary nervous excitement, and when one such exciting influence has had its effect on them, they are ready for another. Religion is with these people a sort of intellectual opium-eating, and there it ends. "There is another sort of man", says Bhagavan Ramakrishna, "who is like the pearl-oyster of the story. The pearl-oyster leaves its bed at the bottom of the sea, and comes up to the surface to catch the rain-water when the star Svâti is in the ascendant. It floats about on the surface of the sea with its shell wide open, until it has succeeded in catching a drop of the rain-water, and then it dives deep down to its sea-bed, and there rests until it has succeeded in fashioning a beautiful pearl out of that rain-drop."

This is indeed the most poetical and forcible way in which the theory of Ishta-Nishtha has ever been put. This Eka-Nishtha or devotion to one ideal is absolutely necessary for the beginner in the practice of religious devotion. He must say with Hanuman in the Râmâyana, "Though I know that the Lord of Shri and the Lord of Jânaki are both manifestations of the same Supreme Being, yet my all in all is the lotus-eyed Râma." Or, as was said by the sage Tulasidâsa, he must say, "Take the sweetness of all, sit with all, take the name of all, say yea, yea, but keep your seat firm." Then, if the devotional aspirant is sincere, out of this little seed will come a gigantic tree like the Indian banyan, sending out branch after branch and root after root to all sides, till it covers the entire field of religion. Thus will the true devotee realise that He who was his own ideal in life is worshipped in all ideals by all sects, under all names, and through all forms.

❑

10

The Method and The Means

In regard to the method and the means of Bhakti Yoga we read in the commentary of Bhagavan Ramanuja on the Vedanta-Sutras: "The attaining of That comes through discrimination, controlling the passions, practice, sacrificial work, purity, strength, and suppression of excessive joy." Viveka or discrimination is, according to Ramanuja, discriminating, among other things, the pure food from the impure. According to him, food becomes impure from three causes: (1) by the nature of the food itself, as in the case of garlic etc.; (2) owing to its coming from wicked and accursed persons; and (3) from physical impurities, such as dirt, or hair, etc. The Shrutis say, When the food is pure, the Sattva element gets purified, and the memory becomes unwavering", and Ramanuja quotes this from the Chhândogya Upanishad.

The question of food has always been one of the most vital with the Bhaktas. Apart from the extravagance into which some of the Bhakti sects have run, there is a great truth underlying this question of food. We must remember that, according to the Sankhya philosophy, the Sattva, Rajas, and Tamas, which in the state of homogeneous equilibrium form the Prakriti, and in the heterogeneous disturbed condition form the universe – are both the substance and the quality of Prakriti. As such they are the materials out of which every human form has been manufactured, and the predominance of the Sattva material is what is absolutely necessary for spiritual development. The materials which we receive through our food into our body-structure go a great way to determine our mental constitution; therefore the food we eat has to be particularly taken care of. However, in this matter, as in others, the fanaticism into which the disciples invariably fall is not to be laid at the door of the masters.

And this discrimination of food is, after all, of secondary importance. The very same passage quoted above is explained by Shankara in his Bhâshya on the Upanishads in a different way by giving an entirely different meaning to the word Âhâra, translated generally as food. According to him, "That which is gathered in is Ahara. The knowledge of the sensations, such as sound etc., is gathered in for the enjoyment of the enjoyer (self); the purification of the knowledge which gathers in the perception of the senses is the purifying of the food (Ahara). The word 'purification-of-food' means the acquiring of the knowledge of sensations untouched by the defects of attachment, aversion, and delusion; such is the meaning. Therefore such knowledge or Ahara being purified, the Sattva material of the possessor it – the internal organ – will become purified, and the Sattva being purified, an unbroken memory of the Infinite One, who has been known in His real nature from scriptures, will result."

These two explanations are apparently conflicting, yet both are true and necessary. The manipulating and controlling of what may be called the finer body, viz the mood, are no doubt higher functions than the controlling of the grosser body of flesh. But the control of the grosser is absolutely necessary to enable one to arrive at the control of the finer. The beginner, therefore, must pay particular attention to all such dietetic rules as have come down from the line of his accredited teachers; but the extravagant, meaningless fanaticism, which has driven religion entirely to the kitchen, as may be noticed in the case of many of our sects, without any hope of the noble truth of that religion ever coming out to the sunlight of spirituality, is a peculiar sort of pure and simple materialism. It is neither Jnâna, nor Bhakti, nor Karma; it is a special kind of lunacy, and those who pin their souls to it are more likely to go to lunatic asylums than to Brahmaloka. So it stands to reason that discrimination in the choice of food is necessary for the attainment of this higher state of mental composition which cannot be easily obtained otherwise.

Controlling the passions is the next thing to be attended to. To restrain the Indriyas (organs) from going towards the objects of the senses, to control them and bring them under the guidance of the will, is the very central virtue in religious culture. Then comes the practice of self-restraint and self-denial. All the immense possibilities of divine realisation in the soul cannot get actualised without struggle and without such practice on the part of the aspiring devotee. "The mind must always think of the Lord." It is very hard at first to compel the mind to think of the Lord always, but with every new effort the power to do so grows stronger in us. "By practice, O son of Kunti, and by non-attachment is it attained", says Shri Krishna in the Gita. And then as to sacrificial work, it is understood that the five great sacrificed [1] (Panchamahâyajna) have to be performed as usual.

Purity is absolutely the basic work, the bed-rock upon which the whole Bhakti-building rests. Cleansing the external body and discriminating the food are both easy, but without internal cleanliness and purity, these external observances are of no value whatsoever. In the list of qualities conducive to purity, as given by Ramanuja, there are enumerated, Satya, truthfulness; Ârjava, sincerity; Dayâ, doing good to others without any gain to one's self; Ahimsâ, not injuring others by thought, word, or deed; Anabhidhyâ, not coveting others' goods, not thinking vain thoughts, and not brooding over injuries received from another. In this list, the one idea that deserves special notice is Ahimsa, non-injury to others. This duty of non-injury is, so to speak, obligatory on us in relation to all beings. As with some, it does not simply mean the non-injuring of human beings and mercilessness towards the lower animals; nor, as with some others, does it mean the protecting of cats and dogs and feeding of ants with sugar — with liberty to injure brother-man in every horrible way! It is remarkable that almost every good idea in this world can be carried to a disgusting extreme. A good practice carried to an extreme and worked in accordance with the letter of the law becomes a positive evil. The stinking monks of certain religious sects, who do not bathe lest the vermin on their bodies should be killed, never think of the discomfort and disease they bring to their fellow human beings. They do not, however, belong to the religion of the Vedas!

The test of Ahimsa is absence of jealousy. Any man may do a good deed or make a good gift on the spur of the moment or under the pressure of some superstition or priestcraft; but the real lover of mankind is he who is jealous of none. The so-called great men of the world may all be seen to become jealous of each other for a small name, for a little fame, and for a few bits of gold. So long as this jealousy exists in a heart, it is far away from the perfection of Ahimsa. The cow does not eat meat, nor does the sheep. Are they great Yogis, great non-injurers (Ahimsakas)? Any fool may abstain from eating this or that; surely that gives him no more distinction than to herbivorous animals. The man who will mercilessly cheat widows and orphans and do the vilest deeds for money is worse than any brute even if he lives entirely on grass. The man whose heart never cherishes even the thought of injury to any one, who rejoices at the prosperity of even his greatest enemy, that man is the Bhakta, he is the Yogi, he is the Guru of all, even though he lives every day of his life on the flesh of swine. Therefore we must always remember that external practices have value only as helps to develop internal purity. It is better to have internal purity alone when minute attention to external observances is not practicable. But woe unto the man and woe unto the nation that forgets the real, internal, spiritual essentials of religion and mechanically clutches with death-like grasp at all external forms and never lets them go. The forms have value only so far as they are expressions of the life within. If they have ceased to express life, crush them out without mercy.

The next means to the attainment of Bhakti Yoga is strength (Anavasâda). "This Atman is not to be attained by the weak", says the Shruti. Both physical weakness and mental weakness are meant here. "The strong, the hardy" are the only fit students. What can puny, little, decrepit things do? They will break to pieces whenever the mysterious forces of the body and mind are even slightly awakened by the practice of any of the Yogas. It is "the young, the healthy, the strong" that can score success. Physical strength, therefore, is absolutely necessary. It is the strong body alone that can bear the shock of reaction resulting from the attempt to control the organs. He who wants to become a Bhakta must be strong, must be healthy. When the miserably weak attempt any of the Yogas, they are likely to get some incurable malady, or they weaken their minds. Voluntarily weakening the body is really no prescription for spiritual enlightenment.

The mentally weak also cannot succeed in attaining the Atman. The person who aspires to be a Bhakta must be cheerful. In the Western world the idea of a religious man is that he never smiles, that a dark cloud must always hang over his face, which, again, must be long drawn with the jaws almost collapsed. People with emaciated bodies and long faces are fit subjects for the physician, they are not Yogis. It is the cheerful mind that is persevering. It is the strong mind that hews its way through a thousand difficulties. And this, the hardest task of all, the cutting of our way out of the net of Maya, is the work reserved only for giant wills.

Yet at the same time excessive mirth should be avoided (Anuddharsha). Excessive mirth makes us unfit for serious thought. It also fritters away the energies of the mind in vain. The stronger the will, the less the yielding to the sway of the emotions. Excessive hilarity is quite as objectionable as too much of sad seriousness, and all religious realisation is possible only when the mind is in a steady, peaceful condition of harmonious equilibrium.

It is thus that one may begin to learn how to love the Lord.

Notes

1. To gods, sages, manes, guests, and all creatures.

❑❑❑

Popular Classic Fiction

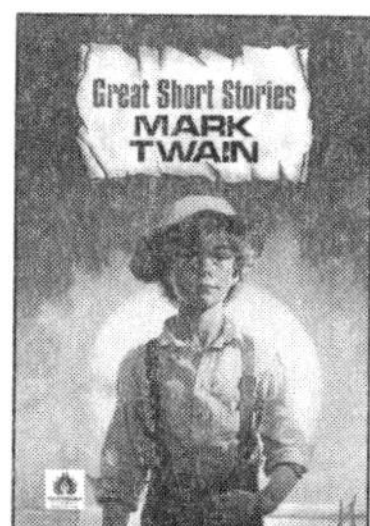

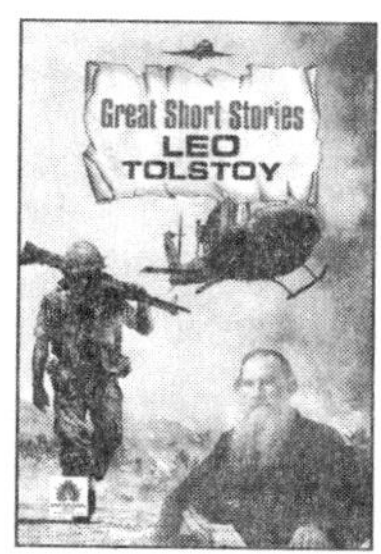

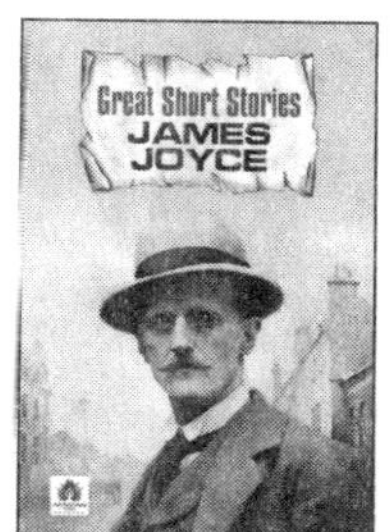

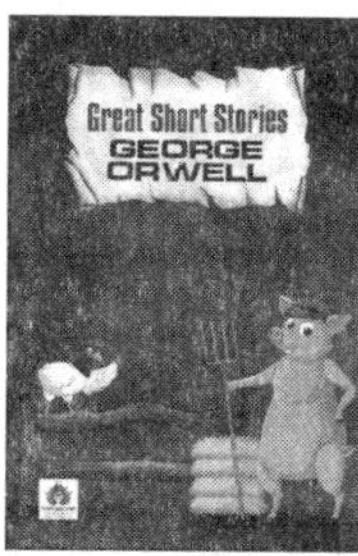

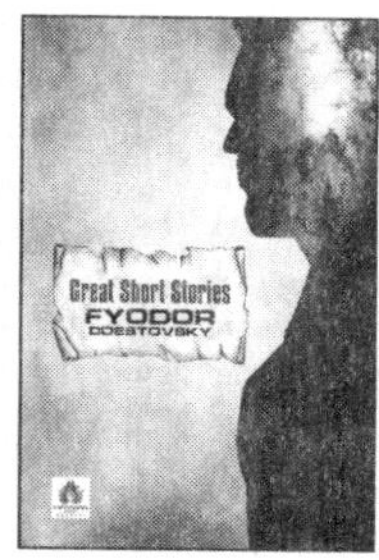

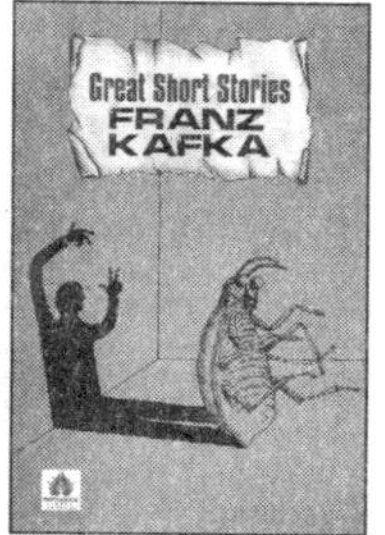

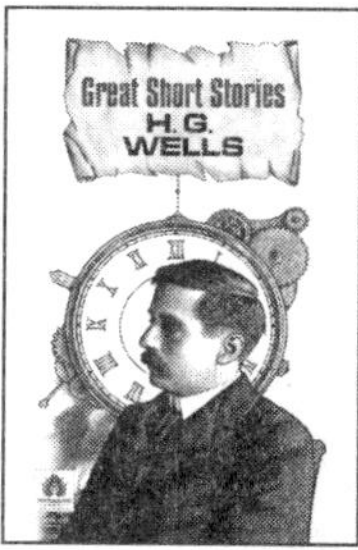

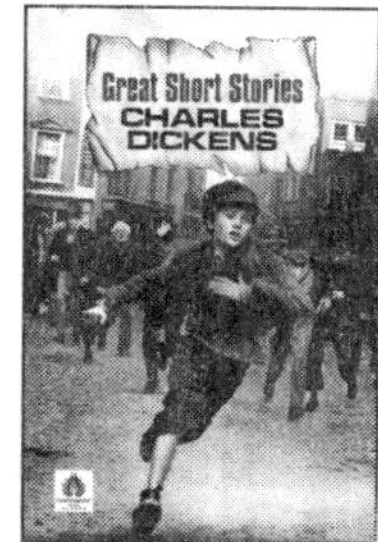

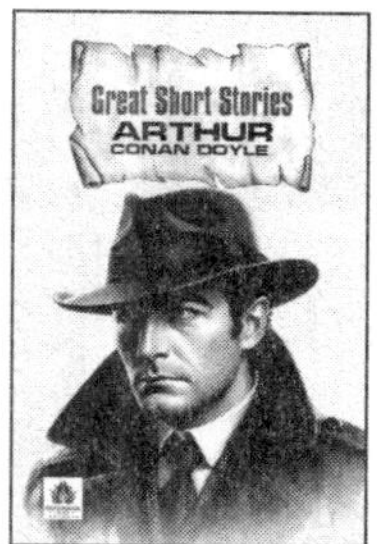

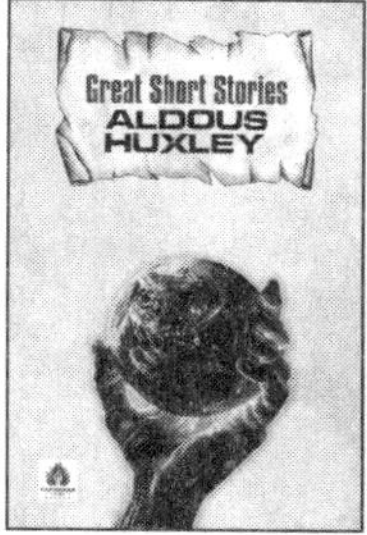

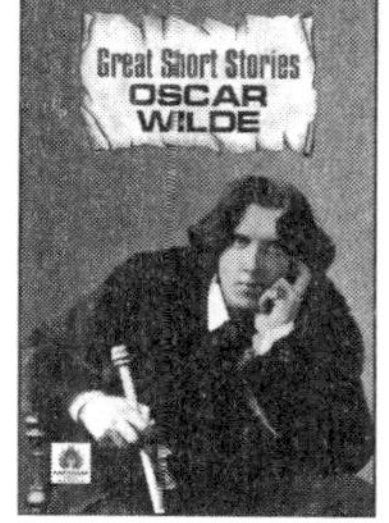